Unisex
Toilet Training

Unisex Toilet Training

Overall Superior, Simpler, Quicker,
Easier, Cleaner and Healthier
Than Standard Toilet Training

Anthony Seymour Browne

Mr. Anthony Seymour Browne
P.O. Box 365
New Rochelle, New York, 10802
U. S. A

Browne, Anthony Seymour
          Unisex Toilet Training

ISBN 978-1492934097

Cover & Book Design by Pub-My-Book.com

Author photo credit: PROphoto Studio, Sheraton Mall, Barbados

Dedication

In1968, I had the insight to toilet train myself to urinate sitting down and enjoy a clean bathroom at home.

Early in 2013, some extraordinary events converge. First, I discovered Taiwan and Sweden have proposals encouraging men to sit down and urinate. Second, I learned why urinating standing up messes up bathrooms are because of the urethra and tip of the penis. Third in 2013 the tools for self-publishing is abundant. Fourth, my Divine Theocratic Education adequately qualifies me to research, write and publish for the benefit of others.

Proverbs 4:18 states. "The path of the righteous ones is like the bright light that is getting lighter and lighter until the day is firmly established." Men sitting down and urinating and producing clean toilets is an idea that is getting brighter and brighter.

Such timing and circumstances are much greater and bigger than me, or any other human. That is why I give all credit and thanks for my unique circumstances and this book, to my all knowing Creator Jehovah, God.

Table of Contents

What is Unisex Toilet Training?

Unisex Toilet Training: This is a new concept the author pioneered for training both toddler boys and girls. Training begins taking the toddler from the diaper stage to sitting down on the potty. Teaching, boy and girl that defecation, stool and urination, pee belong in the, potty. The next step is using a toilet training chair, and boy and girl again is sitting down to have a bowel movement (BM) and also to pee. The last step is using the same sitting posture for the adult toilet. As a result, this new one-step training completely eliminates the time consuming and unhealthy extra step in standard toilet training for a boy, teaching him to stand up and pee. The sitting method is the same for toddler boy and girl. Hence, the appropriate name, Unisex Toilet Training.

Unisex Toilet Training

There is a universal issue where males' public toilets are filthy. The cause is men standing up to urinate. Some countries have proposals encouraging men to sit down to urinate in public toilets.

However, every year millions of little boys worldwide learn to stand up and urinate. It is from this training why men stand up to urinate. The wise King Solomon wrote under inspiration: "Teach a child to choose the right path, and when he is older he will remain upon it." Proverbs 22:6 -- The Living Bible.

That is why; unisex toilet training highlights and addresses the boot-camp and training ground for men standing up to urinate. We must go up stream where they are jumping off. Standard boys' toilet training is where they are jumping off, and the training perpetuates fifthly unsanitary toilets.

This new training eliminates those problems because the new unisex toilet training is overall superior because it is simpler, quicker, easier, cleaner and healthier than standard toilet training.

Toilet Training Boys and Girls

Unisex toilet training begins with taking boys and girls from diapers to sitting down on the potty. This teaches excrement and urine belongs in the potty and usually comes together. As a result, a toddler associates the call of nature with the potty and also with sitting down on the potty.

This feels normal to both sexes and simplifies potty training regardless of gender. This first step of unisex toilet training is the same as traditional toilet training.

The next step in unisex toilet training is teaching boy and girl to sit down on a toilet training seat. When the toddler understands and is comfortable with the training seat then it is time to start using the home toilet.

Mom teaches three steps:

1. Train boy/girl to sit down on the potty to stool and to pee

2. Train boy/girl to sit down on the training seat to stool and to pee

3. Train boy/girl to sit down on the home toilet to stool and to pee

At this stage, Mom successfully provides unisex toilet training for boy and girl.

Those, skills are safe and sanitary bowel and urine elimination that continues throughout the child's life. Let us look at training and the concept of gender.

Concept of Gender

A child's brain receives input from the environment. A key input is the concept of gender for the boy and girl. This essential input begins between two and a half to three years, when both boys and girls show interests in the concept of gender. Boys start to follow fathers and older brother(s), and girls start to follow mothers and older sister(s), and this contributes to the child's development. That is why; signals the parents send to toddlers must be consistent.

Parents Must Send Consistent Signals

In unisex toilet training parents send consistent signals when Mum and Dad sit down for bowel movement and also sit down to urinate. Let us illustrate. What happens if, Mum sits down to pee and sits down to have a bowel movement, but Dad stands up to pee and sits down to have a bowel movement? The parents send conflicting signals to their toddlers.

A toddler's healthy active, inquisitive mind tries to figure out why Mummy sits down on the toilet and why Daddy sits down sometimes and stands up sometimes. This confuses both boy and girl. As a result, they do not know which parent to imitate and perhaps allegiance becomes divided.

On the other hand, when parents are in unity of mind and purpose in unisex toilet training, it speeds up toilet training. In addition, both parents sitting down prevent confusion. Like, a boy or girl, imitating the parent of the opposite sex, action that slows training and produces accidents and makes a mess in the bathroom.

How Parents Achieve Unity of Purpose

How can parents achieve unity of purpose in toilet training? They MUST have an open discussion on child rearing. It is best to do so, long before an offspring arrives. In fact, this is prudent even before a couple gets married. Why so?

What if both prospective mates have extremely strong and opposite opinions on child rearing? Could they produce a healthy environment, for a child's toilet training without conflicts and tug of wars?

Remember, a child's correct time-table for input is during the formative years and is also the most advantageous for the best results.

Why is such a discussion of utmost importance? The activity of going to the bathroom occurs regularly and not occasionally. Therefore, parents and child often come face-to-face with this issue. That is why; the subject of how parents will toilet train their child deserves serious consideration.

For that exact reason, it is wise if a female knows where her prospective partner literally sits, or stands on this issue. Especially if, she hates smelly urine odors in the bathroom, and also hates cleaning it up.

A Good Idea

Here is a good idea. If a prospective husband, or partner, stands up to urinate. He is not a lost cause he needs retraining; so inform him about the sequel to this book by the same Author. It educates males on the exact topic. The title, "Unisex Toilet Retraining: Urinating Sitting Down Produces Clean Toilets. Urinating Standing Up Creates Smelly Filthy Unsanitary Toilets." The male will see the how to, and the many benefits and the female will be happy with the results.

The conclusion of the matter is, parents must have unity regarding toilet training and send the proper signals to their toddler(s). The best way to do so is leading by example and using the home unisex toilet in a unisex manner. That is, both parents sitting down to pee and also sitting down to have a bowel movement. The toddler observes the parents and benefits from teaching and also proper example. In fact, such should be a family affair if, older siblings and other relatives share the same house.

Does it Take Longer to Potty Train Boys Than Girls?

Does it take longer to potty train boys than girls? The child-rearing experts say, **YES** and add: "although no one seems to know just why." These experts provide three possible reasons.

The first reason, "this may be at least partially because Moms are the primary toilet trainers in a family. Boys without a male role model to imitate in the bathroom may take a little longer to get the idea while girls have the advantage of observing someone with the, same equipment."

Same Posture and Same Example

What is important is the same posture and the same example, not the same equipment. What is this same equipment a little girl observes? What she sees is Mum's posture sitting down on the toilet is that not true? So then, if a little boy observes his primary toilet trainer, his mother sitting down, he will also desire to sit down.

Conversely, if a little girl sees her Dad standing up to urinate, she will also desire to imitate him and stand up to urinate. In this case, it is certainly the posture and not the same equipment.

This is the very essence of unisex toilet training: The, parents sitting down when they are peeing, and also sitting down when having a bowel movement. Consequently, this new teaching puts an end to the same equipment idea because same posture and same example are what matters most.

The second reason, "boys tend to need more time than girls might be because learning to pee in a potty is a two-step process. First they learn to do it sitting down, and then they have to master standing up."

The third reason, "boys usually develop slower than girls."

The second and the third reasons make a strong case for boys sitting down to urinate. So let us go there.

Powerful Reasons for Boys Urinating Sitting Down

The powerful reasons for boys urinating sitting down are evident when we consider five points.

Point number one: since the boy knows how to sit down and urinate why change to a two-step method, what are the benefits? Change to a child's routine produces setbacks.

Point number two: the experts agree boys develop slower than girls. So why add extra training after boys master how to pee and poo sitting down?

Point number three: the extra training is an additional handicap for the slower learner. Plus, the two-step system WILL make toilet training for boys longer.

Point number four: the standard toilet extra training provides an inherent disadvantage to boys and a big advantage to girls.

Point number five: it is a fact standing up and urinating produces messy toilets.

Five powerful reasons for training boys the method of urinating sitting down, agreed?

Girls and Boys Follow Same Routine

The new unisex toilet training girls and boys follow the same routine. This is the notable difference. In standard toilet training girls continue to sit down, but boys change.

For example, girls continue urinating sitting down and have a clean, healthy method of peeing. On the other hand, boys the slower learners, change to a toilet training regime that is quite opposite. Standing up and peeing instead of sitting down and peeing. Training, that is traumatic and produces a mess.

What are also astounding, parents and experts wonder why girls continue to do better at school than boys. Could it be the difference in toilet training of boys and their early experiences? Self-inflicted wounds from perceived failure and the trauma of missing the potty, and also, messing up the bathroom?

Girls do not have such experiences because their toilet training is simple and also straightforward. Happily, the new unisex toilet training levels the playing field. Both boys and girls follow the same routine. This benefits both mother and child. Because, it gets rid of their traumatic experiences mother teaching and boy learning to pee standing up.

Unisex Toilet Training

Compare Urinal and Home Toilet

If we compare a urinal and a home toilet bowl on design and function. Sitting down for a bowel movement and sitting down for urinating becomes the obvious choice. The design of a urinal is for males to stand up to urinate in public places. On the other hand, the design of a home toilet is for defecation and not urination.

Why is that distinction beneficial? The urinal has a back-splash and a wall. Yet, the toilet floor and surrounding area get splatters, spills and sprays; when persons stand up and urinate, whether male or female. Therefore, parents should discourage girls who want to pee standing up.

The fact is, standing up to urinate at home, could not have a different outcome than standing up at a urinal. Remember your home toilet design is for sitting down. So if, persons stand up to urinate at home, where are the back-splash and the wall? With a raised toilet seat: the seat, the lid, the hinges and the rim become substitutes for the back-splash, and wall of the urinal and catches the urine that goes astray.

It is true; a boy will have small amounts of urine. Although that is so, small amounts of urine such as tiny droplets, little squirts and delicate sprays, produce excellent growth medium for bacteria. Urine waste breaks down and infects every place urine lands, with smelly urine odor. This creates an unsanitary toilet and a hygienic disaster.

Public urinals are filthy although specifically designed for standing-up and urinating. Therefore, it is reasonable to conclude a little boy standing up and urinating at home with a toilet bowl will also produce a mess.

A loving mother would not teach her toddler son something he will not be able to do, would she? Getting his urine consistently into the toilet is beyond his natural ability. So it frustrates him. That is exactly what teaching a boy the method of standing up and urinating does to him.

Home Toilet Without a Back-splash

The home toilet does not have a back-splash to catch any stray squirts, like a urinal. Plus the toilet bowl comes with a standard height.

That is why, in the home the unisex toilet training, sitting down and urinating is the cleaner method. It ensures the toilet seat is always down and ready for use by the other person, whether male or female. Furthermore, there are no urine spills or odors, because of the right use of the home toilet equipment.

Home Toilet Equipment Right Use

The home toilet equipment right use is sitting down. That is the purpose of the design. A toilet consists of a seat that is a hinged unit and a lid, and they attach to the toilet bowl. The lid covers the toilet when it is not in use.

In the home, both males and females use the same toilet. Consequently, the home toilet functions as a unisex toilet. Since it is a unisex toilet, mothers should train both boys and girls to use it in a unisex manner, sitting down on the toilet to poo and to pee. That is the right use of the home toilet equipment. This brings us to this powerful topic about the home toilet equipment and the wrong use.

Home Toilet Equipment Wrong Use

The home toilet equipment usually consists of the wrong use. Although, the design is for sitting down, some persons use it for standing up and urinating into the bowl. This is the wrong use for the home toilet equipment and persons should not stand to use it as a urinal, since it is not.

Unisex Toilet Training

Toddler Toilet Training Equipment

The first equipment in toilet training toddler boys and girls is a regular potty. This trains boys and girls, to sit down on the potty, to poo and pee and continues until the toddler is comfortable using the potty.

When the child's behavior indicates that they understand and identify the potty and associate it with the call of nature. Then it is time to consider the next unisex training equipment, which is a child-size seat. This is a child-sized adapter toilet seat, and it attaches to the regular adult home toilet.

In some cases, there is alternative new equipment with the child toilet seat already assembled onto the adult toilet seat by the manufacturer.

Toddler, Step-up Equipment Device

Another practical unisex, toddler equipment is a step-up device. Here is why. The adult home toilet and seat combination come in a standard size. This is usually too high for a toddler to reach. So the step-up device allows him/her to climb on to the adult toilet seat.

After they learn how to climb and sit on the adult toilet seat, toilet training is almost complete in unisex toilet training because Mom teaches what she knows.

Mom Teaches What She Knows

Unisex toilet training allows Mom to teach what she knows, which is how to sit-down to urinate and also sit-down to defecate. This makes toilet training less confusing for both Mum and her little boy or girl. Both gender models Mum and identifies and relates to what they observe their primary toilet trainer doing when she uses the bathroom.

Plus, sitting-down is cleaner as it prevents mess and continuous clean-up and extra work. A busy mother has more time for herself and other family members. When Mom teaches what she knows.

A First Time, Mom

Unisex toilet training provides many benefits for the first time Mom. For example, the prospect of toilet training a child often terrifies a first time mom. She fears she lacks previous experience. However, if her first child is a girl, she feels that she knows how to toilet train her little girl. Just simply teach her what she; the Mum does when she uses the bathroom.

On the other hand, when her first child is a boy, she feels overwhelm and does not know where to begin with her little one of the opposite sex.

This is exactly why unisex toilet training is ideal for and benefits the first time mother. She already knows how to sit down on the toilet for a bowel movement and also for urination. Well, that is what she teaches, either a boy or a girl in unisex toilet training.

The standard toilet training makes it difficult for a female to toilet train a boy. The unfamiliar and time consuming second step, of urinating standing up. Unisex toilet training eliminates that second step and simplifies the teaching process so that Mom can teach a boy what she knows and does. In addition, unisex toilet training is also ideal for professional women.

Ideal, For Professional Women

Unisex toilet training is ideal for professional women. For example, sometimes a career woman takes time off to fulfill her desire to be a mother. To, have a child, or children and then return to the work force after toilet training.

As a result, the professional woman seeks the quickest toilet training method. Research shows standard toilet training for boys and girls vary, not only in method, but more importantly, in the time spent in toilet training.

Professional women want to choose the safest and fastest method to toilet train. The traditional boy's toilet training involves extra training. Unisex toilet training is not like that because it is a one-step training method for both boy and girl.

This new training provides a fast-track for siblings of the same sex, and also for siblings of the opposite sex to teach and to learn from each other. This expedites the toilet training process and allows professional women to accomplish both goals: To fulfill her desire to be a mother and also quickly return to her career.

That is why unisex toilet training is ideal for the professional woman because; it is simpler, quicker, easier, cleaner and healthier than standard toilet training.

Easy For Single Mothers

Toilet training a boy was a difficult task for single mothers, but now with unisex toilet training a boy, is easy for single mothers. How so? A Mom's first issue is getting her little boy or girl, out of diapers and sitting down on the potty. What is interesting, sitting down on the potty and the toilet is Mom's main task in unsex toilet training, because this new training solves the single mother and the male role model issue.

Solves The Role Model Issue

Unisex toilet training solves the role model issue. In standard toilet training for boys' the experts suggests single mothers get a suitable male role model. "Having a readily available male role model is the key so arrange for Dad, an uncle, an older brother, or a good family friend to do the honors." The honors of teaching her son how to pee standing up.

Unisex Toilet Training

Unisex toilet training gets rid of a single mother's challenge in that regard. She does not need role models with their poor urine elimination habit teach her son their unhealthy method. Please note, crucial information on toilet training boys are under the topics: "The Boy and Gender-specifics," and also, "Teach Boy to Wipe Penis After He Urinates." Please pay close attention to them.

The good news is the difficulties of a single Mom toilet training a boy are a thing of the past. Unisex toilet training empowers the single mother to toilet train her little son. As a result, she spends less time toilet training and cleaning the toilet seat, and bowl and bathroom floor and have more time for her other important activities.

How to Handle Caregivers

How, to handle caregivers is vital with unisex toilet training. Caregivers should follow the same routine as that of the mother. Young children are creatures of routine, and any change to a usual program is likely to cause setbacks.

Therefore, it is necessary Mom informs the caregivers how she is training her son, to sit down to pee. Then suggests they follow the same method in order to prevent confusion and inconsistent toilet training and setbacks.

The caregivers are usually grandparents, babysitters, nannies, friends, in-laws and daycare providers. These will have their opinions and ideas, about this new unisex toilet training and may even express those feelings.

Please do not become overly annoyed with them. It is best to consider, they mean well and thank them for expressing how they feel. Then politely explain after serious thought, it is in the child's best interest. State the many benefits and why it is superior to the standard training method. As a result, it is beneficial for them to cooperate with this new training.

The self-assurance, the confidence of knowing the value of one's own ideas and opinions are a key factor. This overrides feelings of pressure by caregivers and educates open-minded ones, to the superior, easier, cleaner and healthier, unisex toilet training.

Boys and Girls Controversial Toilet Training Issues

What are boys and girls controversial toilet training issues? First is when to start the toilet training. Second is how to toilet train a boy. Let us start with when to start toilet training. The consensus varies regarding the age at which to start toilet training boys and girls.

There are many articles on readiness and those articles list various signals.

In all the articles, one key point repeats like a refrain, or a mantra. "A mother is the best person to decide when to start toilet training. She knows her child and observes her child's habits and signals. Therefore, she can best determine when her child is ready for toilet training."

Unisex Toilet Training

This indicates the importance and the value of keen observation and awareness in the day-to-day changes and the behavior of toddlers. Otherwise, a mother may attempt to start to toilet train before the child is ready, and the child WILL resist the toilet training.

The best way to avoid the trap of starting toilet training before the child is ready. Resist depending on preset time tables for starting toilet training using a one-size fits all method. A mother must make judgment calls on the basis of her own child's ability and personality.

Mother Has a Choice

As we see a mother has a choice, when to start toilet training. She also has a choice on the method of toilet training for her girl and boy. There is seldom an issue training a girl. The standard choice is sitting down for a bowel movement (BM) and also sitting down for urinating.

In the case of a boy, there are two choices. The boy continues sitting down when having a bowel movement (BM) and also sitting down for urinating. The other choice is the extra toilet training teaching him urinating standing up.

So a mother's decision becomes easy if, she considers these essential facts. When sitting down on the potty, did her little boy miss the potty with his pee? When sitting down on the training toilet seat, did he miss the toilet bowl with his pee? A mother would answer he did not, and that is correct.

Since her son associates sitting down with bowel movement and peeing and he is doing both without mishaps. What are the benefits for changing him to peeing standing up?

Changing a boy to peeing standing up is a new skill. Not only new, it also presents certain difficulties for a toddler. For example, Little Johnny must immediately and accurately identify whether his call of nature is to poo or to pee and instantly take the appropriate action.

Those distinctions are subtle and are often difficult for adults to identify. Imagine, how much more so, for small boys. As a result, boys usually have many accidents wetting their pants and putting excrement in their pants. With so many negative issues, a mother's decision is easy. What are the valid reasons for training a boy to stand up to pee? Giving him a tough task and also giving the mother an eighteen year project?

Mothers' Eighteen Year Project And The Sad Legacy

When, a mother starts training her little boy urinating standing up she undertakes an eighteen year urine cleaning project and a sad legacy. Eighteen years are about the time her son lives at home.

The child-rearing experts make sure they include this stern warning to mothers when recommending teaching a boy to stand up and pee. "It is messy so be prepared to clean up urine." Mothers think this cleaning is only during his training, but the cleaning of a boy's mess is much longer. It is for as long as he remains at home.

What is also disturbing is the sad legacy. He leaves as a young adult and continues his awful habit someplace else and becomes another woman's problem.

Child-rearing Experts Experience

Would child-rearing experts own experience make them aware of the legacy of males urinating standing up? Most certainly! A male's penis and urethra have similar anatomy and function. Therefore, the male experts have the same common experiences as other males. If, they are urinating standing up. Again, tradition is the main reason men experts favor boys standing up and urinating.

What about the female child-rearing experts? Unless, they grew up in an all females home, they also have private knowledge. They know the experiences of male relatives at home; father and brother and spouse and male partner.

That is the child-rearing experts' personal experience, what about their position on still endorsing standing up and urinating.

Child-rearing Experts Position

The child-rearing experts' position may emanate from two points. First, the idea of a theory: but, "We must not reject a theory that we do not like if the experimental evidence supports it."__ Physics Bulletin, Volume 31, 1980, page 138.

Urinating standing up and the results have well-substantiated proof and astounding evidence, worldwide. Plus, the comprehensive research study by Taiwan's **Environmental Protection Administration (EPA)**. This review of 100,000 **inspections of public toilets is a large** population and the conclusions are significant and moves urinating sitting down beyond a theory.

Second, child-rearing experts are waiting the renowned establishments of academia and science endorsement. The child-rearing experts own personal experience should be compelling and sufficient for accepting and endorsing urinating sitting down.

The same is also true for members of the governing establishments in academia and science. They are also aware of, and experience the same challenges and issues when urinating in the standing position.

Unisex Toilet Training, Easier For Mom and Siblings

Unisex toilet training is easier for Mom and for siblings. Remember, whether the first child is a boy or girl they sit down on the potty to poo and also to pee. Please think about these key facts.

The first child trains in the one-step method and toilet training become easier for the second child regardless of which sex comes along afterward.

It is true some mothers have another child as soon as one year, and some mothers have the next child two to five years or more, later. Whatever the interval, unisex toilet training, makes it easier for mother and child. Let us illustrate this fact with a girl as her first child.

The First Child is a Girl

In this scenario, the first child is a girl. Mom teaches her to sit down for both the bowel movement and also the urination. What if the second child is a boy? He imitates what his older sibling does and also sits down on the toilet.

Best of all, he has fun as he imitates the older child. This provides a natural learning process, without urgings from the mother. As a matter of fact, the second child is eager to sit down, just like his older sister.

So Mom gets unsolicited help from her first child, the girl, and Mom allows the boy to sit down. Thus, his potty training becomes easier because he copies his older sister.

To demonstrate how flexible and beneficial this new unisex toilet training is for the first time parent. We switch the birth sequence and child arrival and look at if a mother's first child is a boy.

The First Child is a Boy

What happens when the first child is a boy, and Mom's second child is a girl? Unisex toilet training is also ideal in this reverse situation. How so? Again, with unisex toilet training the little boy sits down for both calls of nature, the bowel movement and also to urinate.

The girl observes her older brother as he sits down to poo and to pee and she also wants to sit down just like her brother. Therefore, as in the first scenario, Mom gets unsolicited help. This time her help is from her first child, the boy.

Clearly, also in this reverse scenario, both mother and younger sibling gets help from the older sibling. This illustrates the versatility of the unisex toilet training, over the standard toilet training for boys. Even better news; this new method also prevents confusing signals and many questions.

Unisex Toilet Training

Prevents Confusing Signals

Unisex toilet training prevents confusing signals when the little boy stands up to pee, and his little sister sits down to pee. Those different postures puzzle little siblings and results in numerous questions. Not only that, but occasionally one gender imitates the other one and creates some challenges for the mother all because of confusing signals.

So in that regard, unisex toilet training works wonders. It is straightforward and easy for Mom and also easy for the other child regardless of gender. They have a role model in the first child. As part of this new training, it is essential to know, the gender-specifics in unisex toilet training for girls and boys.

The Girl and Gender-specifics

The girl(s) gender-specifics in unisex toilet training is vital and understandable. In addition, also critical, so please pay careful attention.

One rule she MUST never violate is when she cleans her anus; allow the same tissue or stool to come into contact with her vagina.

This strict rule prevents infection. So please teach her to wipe from the front, her vagina, to back, her anus; in order to avoid bacteria from her anus to come into contact with her vagina.

Also teach her to pat her vagina with tissue after she pees. This practice dries the area.

Those are gender-specifics in unisex toilet training for a girl.

The Boy and Gender-specifics

What are the gender-specifics in unisex toilet training for a boy? What is new is this. He sits down to pee, and when he finishes he takes toilet tissue and wipes the tip of his penis.

The common practice is when he has a bowel movement he wipes his anus when he finishes. However, it is normal to have a bowel movement and also pee at the same time. One rule he should always follow is: first wipe his penis and then his anus. Never clean his anus first and then his penis. Again, this precaution is to prevent bacteria from his anus to come into contact with his penis.

So the health factor is the same as with a little girl. Matter from the anus should never come into contact with any other area of the body. More now on the new practice for a little boy, wiping the penis rather than shaking the penis.

Teach Boy to Wipe Penis After He Urinates

Teach the little boy to wipe his penis after he urinates. This replaces the horrible habit to shake his penis. Why, this new training? Shaking the penis after urinating is one of the foremost ways to get spots and sprays and urine deposits on the floor, wall, toilet seat and bowl.

So teaching him to wipe the penis is a lasting legacy to a cleaner bathroom.

This skill serves him well later in his adult years and eliminates the need for toilet retraining as an adult. Unisex Toilet Retraining for those who stand up to urinate, the carryover from standard toilet training for, boys.

Those are the key gender-specifics in unisex toilet training for both boys and girls.

Unisex Toilet Training

Multiple Births and Mixed Genders

Unisex toilet training is ideal for mothers of multiple births with mixed genders. There is much joy expecting twins, the most common of the multiple births and discovering the twins are a girl and a boy. What exciting news having a child of each gender at the same birth! One thing is sure unisex toilet training makes the mother's job easy.

How is that so? Well, potty training is the same for the boy and girl. Therefore, it is easier for Mom and also easier for both toddlers as the toddlers observe similar habits. This allows the quicker learner of the twins, to show by example and also help the slower learner. The best teaching method is imitation.

Mom Saves Time, And Extra Work And Frustration

With unisex toilet training Mom saves time and extra work and frustration.

In the case of mixed twins, teaching her girl one method and her boy another method. Mom also avoids answering questions why, one sibling's potty training is different from the other.

Since, unisex toilet training eliminates two different set of instructions it is certainly less draining on a mother, who is perhaps terribly exhausted caring for her twins.

One thing is sure she will not have to clean-up urine from her little boy during his toilet training. This equalizes the toilet training and also avoids an inherent tendency to favor the girl over the boy, because of the extra work he causes during toilet training.

So without a doubt, unisex toilet training makes it easier and simpler and faster to toilet train mixed twins.

Important Information For Females On Fertility Drugs

This is important information for females on fertility medication, or fertility drugs. The process of "In vitro fertilization or IVF the egg fertilizes by sperm outside the body, of the female.

"Research shows that approximately 35 percent of multiple pregnancies, more than one child, oftentimes results from using fertility treatments. It is not unusual to have multiples of twins, two children and triplets, three children. In the United States of

America, multiple birth of twins account for 95 percent of multiple pregnancies." Source: March of Dimes website.

This is pertinent information for females taking fertility enhancement treatment. These may need to unisex toilet train their children and especially, in the case of multiple births with mixed genders.

Unisex Toilet Training

A Basic Home Coeducation

Unisex toilet training is a basic home coeducation. History shows the home is often the first place where coeducational, or co-ed, of mixed-sex education began. Parents are the ones responsible for educating and training their children.

Long, before older institutions of higher learning for the male sex. Or, even before the mid-twentieth century of single-sex education and single-gender education, where male and female students attend separate classes.

What was the basis for single-sex education in many cultures? In many parts of the world; it was due primarily to tradition and to a lesser extent, religion. The same pattern holds true today, regarding toilet training.

Unisex Toilet Training

For example, there were several changes in toilet training methods over the last 40 years. Yet, the old standard practice, teaching, boys to urinate standing up in the home remains the same.

What is the reason? One word is tradition. That is why pediatricians and the American Academy of Pediatrics still recommend teaching a boy standing up and urinating.

Again, since parents are primarily responsible for educating and training their children, unisex toilet training follows this same pattern. Parents must learn from the Baby Boomers experience.

The Baby Boomers Experience

The Baby Boomers experience provides a lesson on how to make a decision on this new unisex toilet training. A Baby Boomer is a person born between 1946 and 1964 in the United States of America. These Baby Boomers are the generation whose parents consulted self-help books and manuals by specialists on child-rearing. For example, a book by Dr. Benjamin Spock, on Child-rearing translated into 42 languages and also had a circulation of almost 50 million copies sold.

Dr. Benjamin Spock later went on record and said that the professionals, including him, were largely to blame. "We didn't realize until it was too late," he admitted, "how our know-it-all attitude was undermining the self- assurance of parents."

APA: A Satisfying Life—Just a Fantasy? — Watchtower ONLINE LIBRARY. (n.d.). Retrieved from http://wol.jw.org/en/wol/d/r1/lp-e/1102000122

Parents Self-assurance

Why, it is necessary to look at unisex toilet training and parent's self-assurance. Review Dr. Spock's candid reflection in the previous paragraph and discover the exact reason. A parent needs the confidence in, and the value of their own ideas and opinions.

Since using the toilet is a daily function throughout one's own life, each parent has a perspective. It is for this exact reason that they know what the right choice for their little boy is.

Also, it is that same ability and judgment why some men sit down at home to urinate. They did not follow someone's argument to sit down, but rather their own unique and distinct perspective. Sometimes, it is after sprays on the toilet seat, or the bathroom floor. A man decides upon sitting down and urinating is the best way to prevent future mess and urine odor for someone else to clean.

That is where unisex toilet training and self-assurance as a parent is vital. No one sees exactly what a parent observes. Plus there is the responsibility to make training decisions, and also, to assist when a child faces peer pressure.

A Boy Faces Peer Pressure

What if a boy faces peer pressure after his successful training in urinating sitting down? His peer pressure may start in the nursery, or kindergarten, or even later. It requires him staying the course and continuing with his healthy sanitary practice sitting down to pee.

It is good to prepare him for the eventuality of peer pressure and explain why he must not follow after the crowd. Otherwise, he may succumb to what others do and say and give up what is best for him in the long run. Please read the following experience, how a little boy stop sitting down and urinating and how his mother regrets the outcome.

"My son is 11 now, but I was a single mother when I was potty training him.

Unisex Toilet Training

I taught him to go sitting down, and as he got older and was exposed to being with other children he learned from them. I honestly wish I would have discouraged this. Is there a rule somewhere that says that men/boys need to pee standing up? Why can't they sit down to keep things clean? My son still misses the toilet at times!" **APA:** As a single mom, how do I teach my son to pee standing up ... (n.d.). Retrieved from http://www.babycenter.com/404_as-a-single-mom-how-do-i-teach-my-son-to-pee-standing-up_70571.bc

As we see this mother regrets her action. The sad outcome, her son continues to mess up the toilet. What could help boys resist peer pressure and stay the course and continue urinating sitting down?

Help A Boy Continue Urinating Sitting Down

How to help a boy to continue urinating sitting down? It starts with education. First, educate him why he sits down to pee and explain why some boys stand up to pee. Also, what the other boys are doing creates a filthy mess. What he is doing produces clean toilets. Second, his parents want the best for him and his future.

Please bring this to his attention. As he mixes with other children, he will observe some children doing things which are dishonest and unclean and unhealthy. In each case, he must choose what he knows is honest and clean and healthy according to his personal values, and that, is the main point.

Unisex Toilet Training

Illustrate, if he had a medical condition such as asthma, hemophilia or a heart condition. Have dietary habits such as vegetarian or religious affiliation, which prohibits certain practices. No matter what he sees other children doing, it would be wisdom on his part not to follow them. Then highlight he must treat sitting down to pee the same way and with the same commitment.

What is vital for both child and parent is, always keep channels of communication open. Ask your son how he is doing and the challenges he is facing. Also, make him feel free to discuss what he is up against. His challenges, his fears and the new things he faces. Such candid open heart reasoning and communicating will help a boy to stay his course and continue urinating sitting down.

Key Differences Between Unisex and Standard Toilet Training

It is beneficial to contrast the key differences between unisex and standard toilet training in purpose, form and origin.

Unisex toilet training is simple one-step training for both boys and girls. Standard toilet training is an unnecessary, difficult two-step method for boys.

Unisex toilet training promotes sitting down and peeing, the safe way, to get urine into the toilet bowl. In contrast, standard toilet training, promotes the false teaching little boys can master their aim with sufficient practice. Get it right and the application serves them for a lifetime. That is not true; otherwise men would have a perfect aim.

Unisex toilet training recognizes the role of the penis and the urethra when males stand up to pee. This makes it highly unlikely for persons urinating standing up without messing the bathrooms and toilets. Standard toilet training promotes a practice that ignores this basic anatomy of the penis.

Unisex toilet training practitioners contributes to clean sanitary toilets and bathrooms. Standard toilet training practitioners create messy toilets and bathrooms.

Unisex toilet training is ideal for the home unisex toilet. Standard toilet training promotes a gender-specific practice that is not suitable for the home unisex toilet.

Unisex toilet training continues the first toilet learning for boys and girls sitting down on the potty. This makes teaching boys easy for Moms, the primary toilet trainers. Standard toilet training complicates matters with a two-step standing up system for boys a teaching difficult for mothers.

Unisex toilet training teaches sanitary and hygienic urine elimination to millions of young boys worldwide. This prevents adding numbers who cause unsanitary toilets and bathrooms. In contrast, standard toilet training, yearly teaches millions of boys to stand up to pee. These become contributors to and maintain unsanitary, smelly toilets and bathrooms and restrooms worldwide.

This is not an exhaustive list but only, the key differences between unisex toilet training, and the standard toilet training.

Nevertheless, it becomes quite clear. Unisex Toilet Training is Overall Superior, Simpler, Quicker, Easier, Cleaner and Healthier than Standard Toilet Training.

Unisex Toilet Training

Glossary

Kindergarten: This describes a variety of different institutions around the world for children ranging in ages from two to seven as part of early childhood education.

Nursery School: Is a school for children between the ages of one and five years. A staff encourages and supervises educational play, as part of early childhood education.

Potty And Potty Training: A potty is a small pot for use as a toilet by an infant or young child. Potty training is teaching how to use the potty and a small size seat for fitting over a toilet seat.

Stool And Pee: Stool: Is feces or body waste, or the act of eliminating that solid waste. Pee is urine and the act of urinating.

Toilet: Is a sanitation fixture, primarily used by humans in the elimination of their solid body waste, excrement and also their liquid waste, urine. Other names are a bathroom, a toilet, a lavatory or a restroom.

Toilet Different Names: The different names bathroom and toilet and lavatory and restroom depend on the country. The British calls the room containing the same fixture a toilet or a loo. In Canada and other areas of North American a bathroom means any room which contains a toilet. In the United States of America, the same facility has the name restroom. Whereas Hong Kong, Australia and Singapore use the word toilet.

Toilet Training: This is the process of training toddlers, both boys and girls, to use the potty and the toilet training seat and the adult toilet.

Unisex: In this definition mean designed for, or suitable to both sexes and not distinguished between male and female. So both genders are able to use it.

Unisex Toilet: This is a toilet or bathroom or restroom or lavatory used by both genders. Therefore, by definition, the home toilet is a unisex toilet and also toilets on buses, trains, airplanes, some restaurants, small businesses and small offices.

Unisex Toilet Training: This is a new name the author developed on training toddler boys and girls. Training begins changing the toddler from the diaper stage to sitting down on the potty. Teaching boy/girl that stool and pee belong in the potty. The next step is a toilet training chair, and boy/girl again is sitting down to have a bowel movement (BM) and also to pee. The last step is using the same sitting posture for the adult toilet. As a result, this new one-step training completely eliminates the time consuming and unhealthy extra step in standard toilet training for a boy, teaching him to stand up and pee. This is the same method for toddler boy/girl. Hence, the appropriate name, Unisex Toilet Training.

Urinal: Is a special toilet males use for urinating. It has the form of a container or simply a wall, with drainage and automatic or manual flushing.

Unisex Toilet Training

About the Author

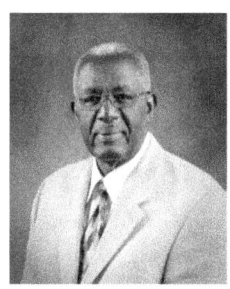 Anthony Seymour Browne has February 11th, 2013 as a memorable day. On that date, he stumbles upon proposals of legislation by Sweden and Taiwan. Encouraging men to sit down to urinate in public toilets, the objective clean toilets.

This interests him; because it is the exact reason why he urinates sitting down. He earnestly researches the topic and discovers the main reasons why a male's urine goes off track. Are because of the urethra, and tip of the penis. This new understanding impresses him because of this fundamental point. When a male stands up and urinates there is the high probability of squirting urine in unintended directions.

He reflects on his own experiences and how standard toilet training was responsible for him squirting urine in the bathroom. Until, in

Unisex Toilet Training

1968, a self-training of urinating sitting down stopped his problem. Anthony, keenly aware the first potty training for toddler girls, and boys are unisex potty training.

Girls continue sitting down through all stages of toilet training and growing as adults and producing clean toilets. Clearly, if boys follow the same routine as girls and continue sitting down they will also grow as adults and similarly produce clean toilets. Those facts provide ideas and title for this book: Unisex Toilet Training, Overall Superior, Simpler, Quicker, Easier, Cleaner and Healthier Than Standard Toilet Training.

Anthony Seymour Browne's two books: unisex toilet training and unisex toilet retraining are both essential for clean toilets and bathrooms without urine odors. The toilet retraining book educates adult males how to have clean toilets and bathrooms. His toilet training book teaches millions of young boys each year the best urine elimination process without causing urine odors. These books are "changing age old traditions and meeting 21st Century global demands:" For, clean bathrooms at home and public unisex toilets and restrooms.

Anthony Seymour Browne was born in Barbados and lived in Montserrat and the U.S.A. Graduate of Bernard M. Baruch College, the City University of New York, with a BBA Degree in Accounting. An Ordained Minister as of June 12, 1993 and he follows Jesus Christ's model. After, 32 years in America Anthony returns to Barbados where he presently resides with his wife, the former Wendy Franklin.